Chapter 1: The Importance of a Balanced Diet

In today's fast-paced world, maintaining a healthy diet can be challenging. With so many food options available, it's easy to fall into unhealthy eating patterns that can negatively impact your health and well-being. However, the benefits of a balanced diet cannot be overstated. Eating a variety of foods that provide essential nutrients can help you feel your best, maintain a healthy weight, and reduce the risk of chronic diseases.

This guide is designed to help you navigate the complexities of maintaining a balanced diet while adhering to a 1500 kcal plan. Whether your goal is to lose weight, maintain your current weight, or simply lead a healthier lifestyle, understanding the fundamentals of nutrition is key. By following a well-structured diet plan, you can ensure that your body gets the right amount of calories, macronutrients, and micronutrients it needs to function optimally.

Understanding Calories

Calories are the units of energy that fuel your body. Every food and drink you consume contains calories, which your body uses to perform basic functions like breathing, digesting food, and maintaining body temperature, as well as more complex activities like exercising. The number of calories you need daily depends on several factors, including your age, gender, activity level, and overall health goals.

For many people, a 1500 kcal diet is an effective and manageable approach to weight management. It provides enough energy to support daily activities while promoting weight loss or maintenance, depending on individual needs. This calorie level is also sufficient to ensure you get all the essential nutrients your body requires without feeling deprived.

Benefits of a 1500 kcal Diet

A 1500 kcal diet offers several advantages:

- *Weight Management*:Consuming 1500 calories a day can help you achieve weight loss, making it ideal for those with goals to reduce body fat in a healthy and sustainable way.

- *Nutrient Balance*: By carefully selecting your foods, you can ensure a good balance of carbohydrates, proteins, and fats, along with essential vitamins and minerals.

- *Sustainable Eating Habits*: Unlike highly restrictive diets, a 1500 kcal plan is more sustainable and less likely to lead to binge eating or feelings of deprivation.

- *Adaptability*: This diet can be easily adjusted for various dietary preferences, including vegetarian, vegan, and gluten-free options.

This guide will walk you through everything you need to know to successfully follow a 1500 kcal diet. From understanding the importance of macronutrients to meal planning and dealing with common challenges, you'll find practical advice and easy-to-follow tips that will help you achieve and maintain a balanced diet.

As you embark on this journey, remember that consistency is key. Small, sustainable changes to your eating habits can lead to long-term success. Let's get started on the path to a healthier, more balanced you!

Chapter 2: Understanding Macronutrients

A well-balanced diet is built on the foundation of macronutrients: carbohydrates, proteins, and fats. These nutrients are essential for providing the energy your body needs to function and perform daily activities. Understanding the role of each macronutrient and how to balance them in a 1500 kcal plan is crucial for maintaining a healthy diet.

Carbohydrates: The Body's Primary Energy Source

Carbohydrates are your body's preferred source of energy. They are broken down into glucose, which fuels everything from your brain to your muscles. Carbohydrates come in two main types: simple and complex.

- *Simple Carbohydrates*: These are sugars found in fruits, milk, and other dairy products. While they provide quick energy, they can also cause rapid spikes and drops in blood sugar levels. Examples include fruit juice, honey, and table sugar.

- *Complex Carbohydrates*: These are found in foods like whole grains, vegetables, and legumes. They are digested more slowly, providing a steady source of energy and helping to maintain stable blood sugar levels. Examples include brown rice, oats, and sweet potatoes.

Balancing Carbohydrates in Your Diet: Aim to get 45-65% of your daily calories from carbohydrates. In a 1500 kcal diet, this equates to about 170-245 grams of carbohydrates per day. Focus on consuming mostly complex carbohydrates, as they provide longer-lasting energy and are rich in fiber, which aids digestion.

Proteins: The Building Blocks of the Body

Proteins are essential for building and repairing tissues, making enzymes and hormones, and supporting immune function. Proteins are made up of amino acids, which are categorized as essential (must be obtained from food) and non-essential (produced by the body).

- *Animal-Based Proteins*: These include meat, poultry, fish, eggs, and dairy products. They provide all the essential amino acids your body needs.

- *Plant-Based Proteins*: These include beans, lentils, tofu, nuts, seeds, and whole grains. While some plant-based proteins may lack one or more essential amino acids, combining different sources (e.g., rice and beans) can provide a complete protein profile.

Balancing Proteins in Your Diet: Aim for 10-35% of your daily calories to come from protein. On a 1500 kcal diet, this translates to about 37-131 grams of protein per day. Including a variety of protein sources, both animal and plant-based, ensures you get all the essential amino acids your body needs.

Fats: Essential for Health

Fats are a crucial part of your diet, despite their bad reputation. They help absorb fat-soluble vitamins (A, D, E, and K), provide energy, and support cell function. Fats come in different forms, and not all fats are created equal.

- *Unsaturated Fats*: These are the "good" fats found in foods like avocados, nuts, seeds, and olive oil. They can help reduce bad cholesterol levels and lower the risk of heart disease.
- *Saturated Fats*: These are found in animal products like butter, cheese, and red meat. While some saturated fats can be part of a healthy diet, excessive intake may increase the risk of heart disease.
- *Trans Fats*: These are artificially created fats found in some processed foods and should be avoided as they can increase bad cholesterol and lower good cholesterol.

Balancing Fats in Your Diet: Aim for 20-35% of your daily calories to come from fats. On a 1500 kcal diet, this is about 33-58 grams of fat per day. Focus on consuming more unsaturated fats and limit saturated and trans fats.

Balancing Macronutrients in a 1500 kcal Plan

A balanced 1500 kcal diet should include:

- *Carbohydrates*: 45-65% of total calories (170-245 grams per day)
- *Proteins*: 10-35% of total calories (37-131 grams per day)

- *Fats*: 20-35% of total calories (33-58 grams per day)

By understanding the role of each macronutrient and how to balance them, you can create a diet that supports your health goals and provides the energy you need throughout the day.

Chapter 3: Micronutrients and Their Role

While macronutrients like carbohydrates, proteins, and fats provide the bulk of your energy needs, micronutrients are equally essential for maintaining optimal health. Micronutrients include vitamins, minerals, and other compounds that play critical roles in everything from bone health to immune function. Understanding how to include these in your 1500 kcal diet is key to achieving a balanced nutritional profile.

Vitamins: Essential for Vital Functions

Vitamins are organic compounds that your body needs in small amounts to function correctly. Each vitamin has specific roles, and a deficiency can lead to various health issues. There are two main types of vitamins:

- *Fat-Soluble Vitamins*: These include vitamins A, D, E, and K, which are stored in the body's fatty tissues and liver. They are absorbed along with fats in your diet, so it's important to consume them with some dietary fat.
- *Vitamin A*: Important for vision, immune function, and skin health. Sources include carrots, sweet potatoes, and spinach.
- *Vitamin D*: Essential for bone health and immune function. It can be synthesized by the skin in sunlight, but is also found in fortified foods and fatty fish.
- *Vitamin E*: Acts as an antioxidant and supports skin health. Found in nuts, seeds, and vegetable oils.

- *Vitamin K*: Crucial for blood clotting and bone health. Found in leafy greens like kale and spinach.
- *Water-Soluble Vitamins*: These include the B-complex vitamins and vitamin C, which are not stored in the body and must be consumed regularly.
- *Vitamin C*: Supports immune function and acts as an antioxidant. Found in citrus fruits, strawberries, and bell peppers.
- *B Vitamins (B1, B2, B3, B6, B12, Folate, etc.)*: These play various roles in energy metabolism, nerve function, and red blood cell formation. Found in whole grains, meat, eggs, dairy, and leafy greens.

Minerals: Building Blocks for Health

Minerals are inorganic elements that are also vital for your body's functions. They are involved in building strong bones and teeth, regulating metabolism, and staying properly hydrated.

- *Calcium*: Essential for bone and teeth health, as well as muscle function. Found in dairy products, fortified plant milks, and leafy greens.
- *Iron*: Crucial for the formation of red blood cells and oxygen transport. Found in red meat, beans, lentils, and fortified cereals.
- *Magnesium*: Important for muscle and nerve function, blood sugar control, and blood pressure regulation. Found in nuts, seeds, and whole grains.
- *Potassium*: Helps maintain normal fluid balance, nerve function, and muscle contractions. Found in bananas, potatoes, and spinach.

- _Zinc_: Supports immune function, wound healing, and DNA synthesis. Found in meat, shellfish, nuts, and seeds.

The Importance of Fiber

While not a vitamin or mineral, fiber is a crucial component of a balanced diet. It aids in digestion, helps maintain stable blood sugar levels, and can lower cholesterol levels. Fiber is found in plant-based foods like fruits, vegetables, whole grains, and legumes.

In a 1500 kcal diet, aim to include 25-30 grams of fiber per day. Eating a variety of fiber-rich foods can support digestive health and keep you feeling full and satisfied.

Hydration: The Role of Water

Water is vital for almost every bodily function, including digestion, nutrient absorption, temperature regulation, and waste removal. Staying hydrated is crucial, especially when following a reduced-calorie diet like the 1500 kcal plan.

- _Daily Intake_: Aim for at least 8 cups (64 ounces) of water per day. You may need more if you're active or live in a hot climate.
- _Hydrating Foods_: Many fruits and vegetables, like cucumbers, watermelon, and oranges, have high water content and can contribute to your hydration.

Balancing Micronutrients in a 1500 kcal Diet

To ensure you're getting a full spectrum of vitamins and minerals, it's important to eat a varied diet rich in whole, unprocessed foods. Focus on including:

- *Colorful Fruits and Vegetables*: Different colors often indicate different vitamins and minerals.
- *Whole Grains*: Provide B vitamins, iron, magnesium, and fiber.
- *Lean Proteins*: Such as poultry, fish, beans, and legumes, which provide essential amino acids and minerals like iron and zinc.
- *Healthy Fats*: Nuts, seeds, and oils that provide fat-soluble vitamins and essential fatty acids.

Chapter 4: Meal Planning Basics

Planning your meals is essential for maintaining a balanced diet, especially when following a specific calorie plan like the 1500 kcal diet. Meal planning helps you make mindful food choices, ensures that you meet your nutritional needs, and keeps you on track to achieve your health goals. In this chapter, we'll explore the basics of building a 1500 kcal meal plan, including portion control, reading nutrition labels, and tips for staying organized.

Building a 1500 kcal Meal Plan

To effectively plan your meals, it's important to understand how to distribute your 1500 calories throughout the day. A balanced meal plan should include breakfast, lunch, dinner, and snacks that together provide all the necessary nutrients while keeping you satisfied.

Here's a basic breakdown of how you might allocate your calories:

- Breakfast: 300-400 kcal
- Lunch: 400-500 kcal
- Dinner: 400-500 kcal
- Snacks: 200-300 kcal

This distribution ensures that you have enough energy throughout the day and avoids large calorie deficits that might leave you feeling hungry or fatigued.

Portion Control: Understanding Serving Sizes

Portion control is a key aspect of maintaining a balanced diet, particularly when following a calorie-restricted plan like 1500 kcal. Understanding serving sizes can help you avoid overeating and ensure that you're consuming the right amount of each food group.

Here are some general guidelines for portion sizes:

- _Proteins_: A portion of meat, poultry, or fish should be about the size of your palm (3-4 ounces).
- _Carbohydrates_: A serving of cooked rice, pasta, or grains should be about the size of your fist (½ cup cooked).
- _Fruits and Vegetables_: Fill half of your plate with fruits and vegetables. A serving of fruit is about the size of a tennis ball, while a serving of cooked vegetables is about ½ cup.
- _Fats_: A portion of healthy fats, like avocado or nuts, should be about the size of your thumb (1 tablespoon or 1 ounce).

Using visual cues like these can help you gauge appropriate portion sizes without the need for measuring cups or scales.

Reading Nutrition Labels

Understanding nutrition labels is an essential skill for meal planning and making informed food choices. Nutrition labels provide information about the calorie content, macronutrient breakdown, and micronutrient content of foods.

Here's how to read a nutrition label effectively:

- _Serving Size_: Always check the serving size first. The nutritional information provided is based on this specific amount.
- _Calories_: Look at the total number of calories per serving to ensure it fits within your daily 1500 kcal plan.
- _Macronutrients_: Check the grams of carbohydrates, proteins, and fats per serving. This helps you balance your macronutrient intake across meals.
- _Fiber_: Aim for foods high in fiber (3 grams or more per serving) to support digestion and help you feel full.
- _Sodium and Sugar_: Monitor your intake of sodium and added sugars. Aim for foods lower in sodium (less than 140 mg per serving) and added sugars.

Being able to decipher nutrition labels will help you make healthier choices, particularly when selecting packaged or processed foods.

Planning and Preparing Your Meals

Effective meal planning involves organizing your meals and snacks in advance, so you're less likely to make impulsive food choices that don't align with your dietary goals.

Here are some tips for successful meal planning:

- _Weekly Planning_: Set aside time each week to plan your meals and snacks. Write down your menu and create a shopping list based on the ingredients you'll need.

- *Batch Cooking*: Prepare larger quantities of food and portion them out for the week. This saves time and ch you always have healthy options available.
- *Use Containers*: Invest in a set of reusable containers to store pre-portioned meals and snacks. This makes it easier to grab a healthy meal when you're short on time.
- *Include Variety:* To avoid monotony and ensure a wide range of nutrients, vary your meals throughout the week. Incorporate different proteins, vegetables, and whole grains.

Staying Organized and On Track

Staying organized is crucial for sticking to your 1500 kcal plan. Here are some additional tips to help you stay on track:

- *Keep a Food Journal*: Track what you eat each day, including portion sizes and calories. This helps you stay accountable and identify any areas where you might need to adjust your diet.
- *Set Reminders*: Use reminders or apps to help you stick to your meal schedule and avoid skipping meals or snacks.
- *Plan for Eating Out*: If you know you'll be dining out, plan your meals accordingly to accommodate the extra calories. Choose dishes that fit within your calorie and macronutrient goals.

By mastering the basics of meal planning, you'll be well-equipped to follow a 1500 kcal diet that is both balanced and satisfying. The next chapter will provide you with a sample 7-day menu to help you get started.

Chapter 5: Sample 1500 kcal Menus

Creating a balanced 1500 kcal meal plan can seem challenging, but with careful planning and a variety of foods, you can enjoy delicious and nutritious meals that keep you full and satisfied. In this chapter, you'll find a sample 7-day meal plan designed to provide balanced nutrition while staying within a 1500 kcal daily limit.

Each day includes three main meals—breakfast, lunch, and dinner—along with one or two snacks. The meals are crafted to provide the right balance of macronutrients (carbohydrates, proteins, and fats) and ensure you meet your micronutrient needs.

Day 1

Breakfast (350 kcal):
- 1 slice of whole-grain toast
- 2 large eggs, scrambled with spinach and tomatoes
- 1 small orange
- 1 cup black coffee or tea

Snack (100 kcal):
- 1 medium apple

Lunch (400 kcal):
- Grilled chicken breast (4 oz)
- 1 cup quinoa
- 1 cup steamed broccoli
- 1 tablespoon olive oil for drizzling

Snack (100 kcal):
* 10 almonds

Dinner (450 kcal):
* Baked salmon (4 oz)
* 1 cup roasted sweet potatoes
* Mixed green salad with 1 tablespoon vinaigrette dressing

Day 2

Breakfast (300 kcal):
* 1 cup oatmeal cooked with water, topped with 1/2 banana and 1 tablespoon almond butter
* 1 cup black coffee or tea

Snack (150 kcal):
* 1 small pear
* 1 ounce low-fat cheese

Lunch (400 kcal):
* Turkey sandwich with 2 slices of whole-grain bread, 3 oz turkey breast, lettuce, tomato, and mustard
* 1 small carrot, sliced

Dinner (450 kcal):
* Stir-fried tofu (4 oz) with mixed vegetables (bell peppers, broccoli, onions) in 1 tablespoon soy sauce
* 1/2 cup brown rice

Day 3

Breakfast (350 kcal):

- Greek yogurt (6 oz) with 1/4 cup granola and 1/2 cup mixed berries
- 1 boiled egg
- Snack (100 kcal):
- 1 small apple

Lunch (400 kcal):
- Grilled shrimp (4 oz) with 1 cup couscous and 1 cup sautéed spinach
- 1 tablespoon olive oil for drizzling

Snack (100 kcal):
- 1/2 cup baby carrots with 2 tablespoons hummus

Dinner (450 kcal):
- Chicken stir-fry (4 oz chicken breast with 1 cup mixed vegetables)
- 1/2 cup cooked brown rice
- 1 tablespoon soy sauce

Day 4

Breakfast (300 kcal):
- Smoothie made with 1 cup unsweetened almond milk, 1/2 banana, 1/2 cup frozen berries, and 1 tablespoon flaxseed
- 1 slice whole-grain toast

Snack (150 kcal):
- 1 small handful of mixed nuts (about 1 oz

Lunch (400 kcal):
- Tuna salad made with 3 oz canned tuna, 1 tablespoon mayonnaise, chopped celery, and mixed greens
- 4 whole-grain crackers

Dinner (450 kcal):
- Baked chicken breast (4 oz) with roasted Brussels sprouts (1 cup) and 1/2 cup mashed potatoes
- 1 tablespoon gravy

Breakfast (350 kcal):
- 1 whole-grain English muffin with 1 tablespoon peanut butter
- 1/2 grapefruit
- 1 cup black coffee or tea

Snack (100 kcal):
- 1 small orange

Lunch (400 kcal):
- Grilled chicken salad with 3 oz chicken breast, mixed greens, cherry tomatoes, cucumber, and 2 tablespoons balsamic vinaigrette

Snack (100 kcal):
- 1 small handful of almonds (about 10)

Dinner (450 kcal):
- Lean beef stir-fry (4 oz beef with 1 cup mixed vegetables)
- 1/2 cup quinoa

Breakfast (300 kcal):
- 1 slice whole-grain toast with avocado (1/4 avocado mashed)

- 1 poached egg
- 1 cup black coffee or tea

Snack (150 kcal):
- 1 small pear
- 1 ounce low-fat cheese

Lunch (400 kcal):
- Grilled salmon (4 oz) with 1 cup mixed green salad, 1/2 cup roasted vegetables, and 1 tablespoon olive oil

Dinner (450 kcal):
- Turkey meatballs (4 oz) with 1/2 cup whole-wheat pasta and 1/2 cup marinara sauce
- Steamed asparagus

Day 7

Breakfast (350 kcal):
- 1 whole-grain waffle topped with 1/4 cup Greek yogurt, 1/4 cup berries, and 1 tablespoon honey
- 1 boiled egg

Snack (100 kcal):
- 1 medium apple

Lunch (400 kcal):
- Chicken and vegetable wrap with 3 oz grilled chicken, 1/2 cup mixed vegetables, and 1 tablespoon hummus in a whole-grain wrap
- 1 small side salad

Snack (100 kcal):
- 1/2 cup mixed berries

Dinner (450 kcal):

- Grilled fish tacos (4 oz white fish, 2 small corn tortillas, shredded cabbage, pico de gallo, and avocado slices)
- 1/2 cup black beans

This 7-day sample menu is designed to help you get started with your 1500 kcal diet, offering a balanced mix of macronutrients, plenty of fruits and vegetables, and satisfying meals. The meals can be adjusted to fit your tastes and dietary needs.

Chapter 6: Tips for Long-Term Success

Maintaining a balanced 1500 kcal diet over the long term requires more than just following a meal plan. It involves making sustainable lifestyle changes, staying motivated, and being adaptable as your needs and circumstances change. This chapter will provide you with practical tips and strategies to help you stick to your 1500 kcal plan and achieve your health goals.

1. Set Realistic Goals

Setting achievable and realistic goals is key to long-term success. Start by defining what you want to accomplish with your 1500 kcal diet. Whether it's weight loss, improved energy levels, or better overall health, having a clear objective will keep you motivated.

- Short-Term Goals: Focus on small, manageable steps, such as eating more vegetables, cutting back on sugary snacks, or sticking to your meal plan for a week.
- Long-Term Goals: Think about your ultimate health and wellness goals. For example, reaching a healthy weight, reducing cholesterol levels, or improving fitness.

Review your goals regularly and adjust them as needed. Celebrate your successes along the way to stay motivated.

2. Monitor Your Progress

Tracking your progress is essential for staying on course. Regularly monitoring your weight, energy levels, and overall well-being can help you identify what's working and where you might need to make changes.

- Food Diary: Keep a daily record of what you eat, including portion sizes and calorie counts. This helps you stay accountable and recognize patterns in your eating habits.
- Physical Measurements: Track changes in your body measurements, such as waist circumference or body fat percentage, in addition to your weight. Sometimes, these metrics provide a better picture of progress than the scale alone.
- Energy and Mood: Pay attention to how you feel throughout the day. Are you more energetic? Do you feel satisfied with your meals? These subjective measures are important indicators of your diet's success.

3. Practice Mindful Eating

Mindful eating involves paying full attention to the experience of eating and enjoying your food without distractions. This practice can help you make healthier choices, avoid overeating, and develop a better relationship with food.

- Eat Slowly: Take your time to chew and savor each bite. This gives your body time to signal when it's full, helping you avoid overeating.
- Avoid Distractions: Try to eat without distractions like watching TV or scrolling through your phone. Focus on the taste, texture, and aroma of your food.

- Listen to Your Body: Learn to recognize your body's hunger and fullness cues. Eat when you're truly hungry, and stop when you feel satisfied, not stuffed.

4. Stay Hydrated

Proper hydration is crucial for overall health and can support your weight management efforts. Sometimes, feelings of hunger can be mistaken for thirst, leading to unnecessary snacking.

- Daily Water Intake: Aim for at least 8 cups (64 ounces) of water per day. You may need more if you're active or live in a hot climate.
- Water-Rich Foods: Include water-rich foods like cucumbers, watermelon, and oranges in your diet. These can help with hydration while adding variety to your meals.
- Limit Sugary Drinks: Cut back on sugary beverages like sodas and juices. These can add empty calories and sabotage your 1500 kcal plan.

5. Be Flexible and Adaptable

Life is unpredictable, and there will be times when sticking to your meal plan is challenging. Being flexible and adaptable is key to long-term success.

- Plan for Social Events: If you have a party or dinner out, plan your meals around it. Choose lighter options earlier in the day to accommodate a higher-calorie meal.
- Healthy Substitutions: Learn how to make healthier swaps in your favorite recipes. For example, use Greek yogurt instead of sour

cream, or whole-grain bread instead of white bread.
- Don't Stress Over Slip-Ups: If you go over your calorie limit or indulge in an unplanned treat, don't get discouraged. One meal won't derail your progress. Get back on track with your next meal.

6. Incorporate Physical Activity

While this guide focuses on diet, incorporating physical activity into your routine can enhance your results and improve overall health. Exercise helps you burn more calories, build muscle, and boost your metabolism.

- Find Activities You Enjoy: Whether it's walking, swimming, yoga, or weightlifting, choose activities that you enjoy and can sustain over time.
- Start Small: If you're new to exercise, start with short, manageable sessions and gradually increase the duration and intensity.
- Consistency Over Intensity: Consistency is more important than intensity. Aim for regular, moderate exercise that fits your lifestyle.

7. Seek Support

Having a support system can make a big difference in your success. Whether it's friends, family, or a professional, having people to encourage and motivate you can help you stay on track.

- Join a Group: Consider joining a group or community that shares similar health goals. Online forums, social media groups, or local clubs can provide support and accountability.
- Work with a Professional: If needed, consult with a dietitian, nutritionist, or health coach who can provide personalized guidance and help you navigate challenges.
- Share Your Journey: Don't be afraid to share your goals and progress with those close to you. Their encouragement can be a powerful motivator.

8. Make It a Lifestyle

The ultimate goal is to make your 1500 kcal diet a sustainable lifestyle rather than a short-term fix. By incorporating the tips in this chapter, you'll develop healthy habits that last a lifetime.

- Focus on Balance: Aim for balance rather than perfection. It's okay to enjoy treats and indulgences in moderation as part of a healthy diet.
- Enjoy the Process: Find joy in preparing meals, trying new recipes, and discovering healthy foods that you love.
- Be Patient: Change takes time, so be patient with yourself. Focus on progress, not perfection, and celebrate every step forward.

With these tips, you'll be well-equipped to maintain your 1500 kcal diet for the long term, helping you achieve and sustain your health and wellness goals.

Chapter 7: Overcoming Common Challenges

Embarking on a 1500 kcal diet is a positive step toward better health, but it's natural to encounter challenges along the way. Whether it's dealing with hunger, staying motivated, or navigating social situations, this chapter will help you overcome common obstacles that may arise as you follow your balanced diet plan.

1. Managing Hunger and Cravings

One of the most common challenges when following a calorie-restricted diet is dealing with hunger and cravings. However, with the right strategies, you can manage these feelings without derailing your progress.

- Eat High-Fiber Foods: Fiber-rich foods like fruits, vegetables, whole grains, and legumes help you feel full longer. Incorporating these into your meals can reduce hunger between meals.
- Include Protein in Every Meal: Protein is more satiating than carbohydrates or fats. Make sure each meal includes a good source of protein, such as lean meats, eggs, tofu, or legumes, to keep hunger at bay.
- Stay Hydrated: Sometimes thirst is mistaken for hunger. Drink water regularly throughout the day, especially before meals, to help control appetite.
- Plan Satisfying Snacks: If you get hungry between meals, have a healthy, low-calorie snack like a small apple with peanut butter or a handful of nuts ready. Planning your snacks helps prevent impulsive eating.

- Mindful Eating Techniques: Practice mindful eating to better understand your hunger cues. Take time to enjoy your food, chew slowly, and avoid distractions while eating. This can help you recognize when you're truly hungry versus when you're eating out of boredom or habit.

2. Staying Motivated Over Time

Maintaining motivation can be challenging, especially as the initial excitement of starting a new diet begins to fade. Here's how to keep your motivation strong:

- _Set Mini-Goals_: Break down your long-term goals into smaller, more achievable milestones. Celebrate each mini-goal reached, such as losing a certain amount of weight or sticking to your plan for a month.

- _Track Your Progress_: Use a journal or an app to record your meals, workouts, and how you feel. Seeing your progress over time can boost motivation and provide insight into what's working.

- _Visualize Success_: Picture yourself achieving your goals, whether it's wearing a favorite outfit, feeling more energetic, or reaching a target weight. Visualization can reinforce your commitment.

- _Find Inspiration_: Follow health and wellness accounts, read success stories, or connect with others who share your goals. Seeing others succeed can inspire you to stay on track.

- _Reward Yourself_: Plan non-food rewards for reaching milestones, like treating yourself to a new book, a spa day, or a fun activity. Rewards give you something to look forward to and celebrate your hard work.

3. Navigating Social Situations

Social events can be challenging when you're following a specific diet. Here are some tips to help you stay on track while enjoying social occasions:

- _Plan Ahead_: If you're going to a restaurant, check the menu online beforehand and choose options that fit your calorie plan. If you're attending a party, eat a healthy snack before you go to avoid overeating.

- _Communicate Your Goals_: Let your friends and family know about your dietary goals. Most people will be supportive and may even accommodate your needs when planning meals or events.

- _Make Smart Choices:_ At buffets or gatherings, fill your plate with healthier options like salads, lean proteins, and vegetables. Limit high-calorie foods like fried items, desserts, and heavy sauces.

- _Practice Portion Control_: If you want to indulge in a treat, practice portion control. Enjoy a small piece of cake or a few bites of a favorite dish rather than a large serving.

- _Don't Be Afraid to Say No_: It's okay to politely decline food or drinks that don't fit into your plan. Remember, your health goals are a priority.

4. Dealing with Plateaus

It's common to hit a plateau where your progress seems to stall. This can be frustrating, but there are ways to overcome it:

- _Reevaluate Your Calorie Intake_: As you lose weight, your body requires fewer calories to maintain its current weight. Consider adjusting your calorie intake slightly if you've been following the same plan for a while.

- _Increase Physical Activity_: Adding more physical activity can help break through a plateau. Try incorporating strength training, which builds muscle and boosts metabolism, along with your regular cardio.

- _Mix Up Your Routine_: Sometimes, your body adapts to a routine, causing progress to slow. Try changing your exercise routine, trying new recipes, or eating different foods to keep your body guessing.

- _Stay Positive_: Plateaus are a normal part of the weight loss journey. Stay positive and focused on your long-term goals. Remember that progress isn't always linear, but every healthy choice brings you closer to your goals.

5. Handling Emotional Eating

Emotional eating, or eating in response to emotions rather than hunger, can sabotage your progress. Learning to manage emotional eating is crucial for long-term success:

- *Identify Triggers:* Pay attention to situations, feelings, or times of day when you're more likely to eat emotionally. Keeping a food journal can help you identify patterns.

- *Find Alternatives*: Develop non-food coping strategies for dealing with emotions. This might include going for a walk, calling a friend, practicing deep breathing, or engaging in a hobby you enjoy.

- *Practice Mindfulness*: Before reaching for food, pause and ask yourself if you're truly hungry. If not, identify what you're feeling and consider how you can address that emotion without food.

- *Seek Support:* If emotional eating is a significant challenge, consider seeking support from a therapist or counselor who specializes in eating behaviors. They can help you develop healthier coping mechanisms.

6. Managing Time and Convenience

In today's busy world, finding time to prepare healthy meals can be challenging. Here's how to manage your time effectively whilo ctioking to your 1500 kcal plan.

- *Meal Prep:* Set aside time each week to plan and prepare your meals. Batch cooking and prepping ingredients in advance can save time during the week and ensure you have healthy meals ready to go.

- *Quick and Healthy Options*: Keep healthy, convenient options on hand for days when you're short on time. Stock your kitchen with items like pre-washed salad greens, canned beans, frozen vegetables, and lean proteins that can be quickly prepared.

- *Healthy Takeout*: If you need to order takeout, choose healthier options like grilled proteins, salads with dressing on the side, or vegetable-based dishes. Be mindful of portion sizes and high-calorie extras.

- *Prioritize Your Health*: Remember that your health is worth the time and effort it takes to plan and prepare meals. Make meal planning and preparation a priority, just like you would with other important tasks.

By addressing these common challenges, you'll be better equipped to maintain your 1500 kcal diet and continue making progress toward your health goals.

Chapter 8: The Role of Exercise in a Balanced Diet

While diet plays a crucial role in achieving and maintaining a healthy weight, exercise is equally important for overall health and well-being. Physical activity not only helps you burn calories but also offers a range of benefits that support your 1500 kcal diet plan. In this chapter, we'll explore the different types of exercise, their benefits, and how to incorporate them into your routine to maximize your results.

1. Benefits of Exercise

Exercise offers numerous benefits that extend beyond weight management. Regular physical activity can enhance your physical and mental health in several ways:

- *Increased Calorie Burn*: Exercise helps you burn calories, which can create a larger calorie deficit when combined with a 1500 kcal diet. This can accelerate weight loss or help maintain weight loss over time.
- *Improved Metabolism*: Strength training and high-intensity workouts can boost your metabolism by increasing muscle mass. Muscle tissue burns more calories at rest than fat tissue, helping you maintain a healthy weight.
- *Enhanced Mood and Mental Health*: Physical activity releases endorphins, which are natural mood lifters. Regular exercise can reduce stress, anxiety, and symptoms of depression, contributing to better mental well-being.

- *Better Sleep*: Exercise can improve sleep quality and help you fall asleep faster. Good sleep is essential for overall health and can support weight management by regulating hunger hormones.
- *Increased Energy Levels*: Regular exercise can improve your cardiovascular health and increase your stamina, leading to higher energy levels throughout the day.
- *Reduced Risk of Chronic Diseases*: Physical activity is linked to a lower risk of chronic diseases such as heart disease, type 2 diabetes, and certain cancers. It also supports healthy blood pressure and cholesterol levels.

2. Types of Exercise

To get the most out of your exercise routine, it's important to include a variety of activities that target different aspects of fitness. Here are the main types of exercise to consider:

- *Cardiovascular (Aerobic) Exercise*: Cardio exercises, such as walking, running, cycling, and swimming, increase your heart rate and improve cardiovascular health. These activities are effective for burning calories and enhancing endurance.

- *Strength Training*: Strength or resistance training involves exercises that build muscle and increase strength. Examples include weightlifting, bodyweight exercises (like push-ups and squats), and resistance band workouts. Strength training boosts metabolism and helps you maintain muscle mass as you lose weight.

- *Flexibility and Mobility Exercises*: Activities like stretching, yoga, and Pilates improve flexibility, mobility, and balance. These exercises can enhance your range of motion, reduce the risk of injury, and promote relaxation.

- *High-Intensity Interval Training (HIIT)*: HIIT involves short bursts of intense exercise followed by brief periods of rest or low-intensity activity. HIIT workouts are efficient and effective for burning calories and improving cardiovascular fitness in a shorter amount of time.

- *Low-Impact Exercise*: For those with joint issues or other physical limitations, low-impact exercises such as swimming, cycling, or using an elliptical machine can provide a good workout without putting too much strain on the body.

3. Creating a Balanced Exercise Routine

A balanced exercise routine includes a mix of the different types of exercises mentioned above. Here's how to create a well-rounded routine that complements your 1500 kcal diet:

- *Cardio*: Aim for at least 150 minutes of moderate-intensity cardio (e.g., brisk walking) or 75 minutes of vigorous-intensity cardio (e.g., running) per week. You can break this down into 30-minute sessions, five days a week.

- *Strength Training*: Include strength training exercises at least two to three times per week. Focus on all major muscle groups, including legs, back, chest, arms, and core. Start with lighter weights and gradually increase as you build strength.

- *Flexibility*: Incorporate flexibility exercises, such as stretching or yoga, at least two to three times per week. These can be done after your workouts or on rest days to improve flexibility and aid recovery.

- *HIIT*: If you're short on time or want to boost your calorie burn, add one to two HIIT sessions per week. These can be as short as 20-30 minutes and can be adapted to your fitness level.

- *Rest and Recovery*: Rest days are crucial for allowing your body to recover and repair. Aim for at least one to two rest days per week, depending on the intensity of your workouts. Active recovery, such as light walking or gentle yoga, can also be beneficial.

4. Staying Motivated to Exercise

Just like with your diet, staying motivated to exercise regularly can be challenging. Here are some strategies to keep you engaged and committed to your fitness routine:

- *Set Specific Goals*: Define clear, achievable fitness goals, such as running a 5K, lifting a certain amount of weight, or completing a specific number of workouts each week. Having a target to work towards can keep you motivated.

- *Track Your Progress*: Use a fitness tracker, app, or journal to monitor your workouts, track your progress, and celebrate your achievements. Seeing how far you've come can boost your motivation.

- *Mix It Up:* Avoid boredom by varying your workouts. Try new activities, change your routine, or join a class. Mixing it up keeps things interesting and challenges your body in different ways.

- *Find a Workout Buddy*: Exercising with a friend or joining a group can make workouts more enjoyable and provide accountability. You're less likely to skip a workout if someone is counting on you.

- *Reward Yourself*: Set up a reward system for meeting your fitness goals. Treat yourself to something special, like new workout gear, a massage, or a fun activity, as a reward for your hard work.

- *Listen to Your Body:* Pay attention to how your body feels during and after exercise. If you're feeling overly fatigued or experiencing pain, it's okay to scale back and give yourself time to recover.

5. Combining Diet and Exercise for Optimal Results

To maximize the benefits of your 1500 kcal diet, it's important to align your exercise routine with your nutritional goals:

- *Pre-Workout Nutrition*: Fuel your workouts with a small snack or meal that includes carbohydrates and protein. This could be a banana with peanut butter, a small smoothie, or a slice of whole-grain toast with avocado. Eating before exercise helps provide energy and supports muscle recovery.

- *Post-Workout Nutrition*: After exercise, replenish your body with a balanced meal that includes protein, carbohydrates, and healthy fats. This helps repair muscles and restore glycogen levels. Good options include a chicken and vegetable stir-fry with brown rice, a turkey sandwich on whole-grain bread, or a protein smoothie with fruit.

- *Adjusting Calorie Intake*: If you're engaging in intense or prolonged exercise, you may need to adjust your calorie intake slightly to ensure you're fueling your body adequately. Consult with a dietitian or nutritionist if you're unsure about how to balance your calorie intake with your exercise routine.

- *Listen to Your Hunger Cues*: Exercise can increase your appetite, so it's important to listen to your hunger cues. Choose nutrient-dense snacks and meals that align with your 1500 kcal plan, and avoid eating out of habit or boredom.

By incorporating regular exercise into your lifestyle, you'll enhance the benefits of your 1500 kcal diet and improve your overall health and well-being.

Chapter 9: Maintaining Your Progress

After investing time and effort into following a 1500 kcal diet and incorporating exercise into your routine, it's essential to focus on maintaining your progress. This chapter will guide you through strategies to sustain your healthy habits long-term, prevent setbacks, and continue enjoying the benefits of your new lifestyle.

1. The Importance of Consistency

Consistency is key when it comes to maintaining your progress. Developing a sustainable routine that fits your lifestyle is crucial for long-term success.

- *Stick to Your Routine*: Once you've found a routine that works for you, try to stick with it. Consistency in your eating habits and exercise routine will help reinforce your new lifestyle as a permanent change rather than a temporary diet.

- *Daily Habits*: Focus on small, daily habits that support your goals. Whether it's drinking enough water, eating a balanced breakfast, or taking a walk after dinner, these habits add up over time and contribute to your overall success.

- *Accountability*: Keep yourself accountable by tracking your progress, setting regular check-ins, or finding an accountability partner who shares similar goals. Knowing someone is there to support you can keep you motivated.

2. Monitoring Your Progress

Regularly monitoring your progress is important to ensure you're staying on track and making any necessary adjustments.

- *Track Your Weight and Measurements*: Regularly weigh yourself or take measurements to monitor changes in your body. However, remember that weight is just one indicator of progress—focus on how you feel and other improvements in your health as well.

- *Journal Your Food Intake*: Keep a food journal to track what you're eating, how much, and when. This can help you identify patterns, such as emotional eating or portion sizes, that may need adjustment.

- *Assess Your Energy Levels*: Pay attention to how your energy levels fluctuate throughout the day. If you notice significant changes, consider evaluating your diet, exercise, and sleep patterns to find the cause.

- *Reflect on Your Mental Health*: Take time to reflect on your mental and emotional well-being. A healthy lifestyle should contribute to your overall happiness and reduce stress, so consider making changes if you're feeling overwhelmed.

3. Dealing with Setbacks

It's natural to experience setbacks along the way, whether it's an indulgent weekend, a missed workout, or a period of stress that affects your habits. The key is to handle setbacks in a way that doesn't derail your progress.

- *Don't Be Too Hard on Yourself:* Remember that setbacks are a normal part of any journey. Rather than focusing on what went wrong, concentrate on getting back on track as soon as possible.

- *Reframe Setbacks as Learning Opportunities*: View any challenges you face as opportunities to learn. Identify what triggered the setback and how you can prevent it in the future.

- *Make Adjustments When Necessary*: If you find that certain strategies aren't working for you, don't be afraid to make adjustments. Your plan should be flexible enough to adapt to your needs and lifestyle changes.

4. Preventing Relapse into Old Habits

Maintaining progress also involves preventing a relapse into old habits that could undermine your success.

- *Identify Triggers*: Be aware of situations, emotions, or environments that might trigger a return to unhealthy habits. Whether it's stress, boredom, or social settings, knowing your triggers can help you avoid them or develop strategies to cope.

- *Stay Mindful of Portions*: Even after reaching your goals, continue to be mindful of portion sizes. It's easy to slip back into old habits, especially with portion distortion being so common in today's society.

- *Keep Learning*: Stay informed about nutrition, fitness, and health. The more you learn, the better equipped you'll be to make informed decisions and resist the temptation to fall back into unhealthy patterns.

5. Celebrating Milestones

Celebrating your achievements is an important part of maintaining your progress. Recognizing how far you've come can motivate you to continue your journey.

- *Acknowledge Your Achievements*: Take time to reflect on what you've accomplished. Whether it's losing weight, improving your fitness, or adopting healthier eating habits, celebrate your success.

- *Reward Yourself*: Consider rewarding yourself when you reach specific milestones. Rewards don't have to involve food—they could be a new piece of clothing, a relaxing day out, or a fun experience you've been looking forward to.

- *Share Your Success*: Sharing your journey with others can be incredibly rewarding. Whether it's with friends, family, or an online community, celebrating your success with others can provide additional motivation and support.

6. Long-Term Health and Wellness

Maintaining your progress isn't just about staying on track with your diet and exercise—it's about embracing a long-term commitment to health and wellness.

- *Focus on Overall Wellness*: Beyond diet and exercise, consider other aspects of wellness, such as mental health, stress management, and sleep. A holistic approach to health will support your long-term success.

- *Set New Goals*: Once you've achieved your initial goals, set new ones to keep yourself challenged and motivated. This could involve trying new forms of exercise, learning more about nutrition, or exploring other areas of health and wellness.

- *Stay Inspired*: Keep finding sources of inspiration to fuel your journey. Whether it's reading success stories, learning from experts, or connecting with like-minded individuals, staying inspired will help you maintain your progress.

As you continue to implement these strategies, you'll be well-equipped to maintain your progress and enjoy the benefits of your 1500 kcal diet and healthy lifestyle for years to come.

Chapter 10: Mindful Eating and Lifestyle Habits

Mindful eating and adopting healthy lifestyle habits are essential components of sustaining a balanced diet and overall well-being. This chapter will explore the principles of mindful eating, how to develop healthy habits, and ways to integrate these practices into your daily life for lasting success.

1. What Is Mindful Eating?

Mindful eating is the practice of being fully present and engaged during meals. It involves paying attention to the food you eat, how it makes you feel, and recognizing your body's hunger and fullness cues.

- *Awareness*: Mindful eating starts with being aware of what and how much you're eating. It involves noticing the flavors, textures, and smells of your food and how it makes you feel before, during, and after eating.

- *Non-Judgmental Observation*: Instead of labeling foods as "good" or "bad," mindful eating encourages you to observe your eating habits without judgment. This approach fosters a healthier relationship with food and reduces guilt or shame associated with eating.

- *Listening to Your Body*: Mindful eating involves tuning into your body's hunger and fullness signals. It encourages you to eat when you're hungry and stop when you're satisfied, rather than eating out of habit or emotion.

- *Slowing Down*: Eating slowly allows you to savor your food and gives your body time to signal when it's full. This can help prevent overeating and improve digestion.

2. Benefits of Mindful Eating

Practicing mindful eating offers several benefits that support your 1500 kcal diet and overall health:

- *Better Portion Control*: By paying attention to hunger and fullness cues, you're more likely to eat appropriate portion sizes, which can help you stay within your calorie goals.

- *Improved Digestion*: Eating slowly and chewing thoroughly aids digestion, allowing your body to absorb nutrients more effectively.

- *Reduced Emotional Eating*: Mindful eating helps you recognize emotional triggers for eating, such as stress or boredom, and develop healthier coping strategies.

- *Increased Enjoyment of Food*: When you eat mindfully, you're more likely to appreciate and enjoy your meals, leading to greater satisfaction and reduced cravings.

- *Enhanced Awareness of Nutritional Needs*: Mindful eating encourages you to pay attention to how different foods make you feel, helping you make choices that align with your nutritional needs and overall well-being.

3. Practicing Mindful Eating

Incorporating mindful eating into your daily routine can be simple and rewarding. Here are some practical tips to get started:

- _Eat Without Distractions_: Avoid eating while watching TV, using your phone, or working. Instead, focus solely on your meal and the experience of eating.

- _Take Small Bites_: Take smaller bites and chew your food thoroughly. This helps you slow down and savor each bite.

- _Pause Between Bites_: Put your fork down between bites and take a moment to breathe and reflect on how the food tastes and how full you feel.

- _Check in with Yourself_: Throughout your meal, check in with your body to assess your hunger and fullness levels. Stop eating when you feel comfortably full, even if there's food left on your plate.

- _Practice Gratitude_: Take a moment before eating to appreciate your food and express gratitude for the nourishment it provides.

4. Developing Healthy Lifestyle Habits

In addition to mindful eating, cultivating healthy lifestyle habits is essential for long-term success. These habits contribute to overall well-being and make it easier to maintain a balanced diet.

- *Establish a Regular Eating Schedule*: Eating at consistent times each day can help regulate your metabolism and prevent overeating. Aim for three balanced meals and one or two healthy snacks, depending on your needs.

- *Stay Hydrated*: Drinking enough water is crucial for overall health and can help prevent overeating by reducing feelings of hunger. Carry a water bottle with you and sip throughout the day.

- *Prioritize Sleep*: Adequate sleep is essential for overall health and can support weight management by regulating hunger hormones. Aim for 7-9 hours of sleep per night and establish a relaxing bedtime routine.

- *Manage Stress*: Chronic stress can lead to emotional eating and weight gain. Practice stress management techniques, such as meditation, deep breathing, or spending time in nature, to support your mental and physical health.

- *Stay Active*: Incorporating regular physical activity into your routine is important for overall health. Find activities you enjoy, whether it's walking, dancing, or yoga, and aim to move your body every day.

5. Integrating Mindfulness and Healthy Habits into Your Life

To successfully integrate mindfulness and healthy habits into your daily life, consider the following strategies:

- *Start Small*: Begin by incorporating one or two mindful eating practices or healthy habits into your routine. Gradually add more as you become comfortable with the changes.

- *Create a Supportive Environment*: Surround yourself with a supportive environment that encourages healthy choices. Keep healthy foods on hand, create a calming eating space, and seek support from friends or family members who share your goals.

- *Set Realistic Expectations*: Remember that change takes time. Be patient with yourself as you develop new habits and focus on progress, not perfection.

- *Practice Self-Compassion*: Be kind to yourself if you encounter setbacks or challenges. Rather than being critical, approach setbacks as opportunities to learn and grow.

- *Reflect Regularly*: Take time to reflect on your progress and how you feel. Regular reflection can help you stay motivated and make adjustments to your routine as needed.

By embracing mindful eating and healthy lifestyle habits, you'll not only support your 1500 kcal diet but also enhance your overall quality of life. These practices will help you maintain balance, prevent burnout, and enjoy a sustainable, healthy lifestyle.

Final Thoughts and Resources

As we conclude this guide on maintaining a balanced diet with a 1500 kcal plan, it's important to reflect on the journey you've embarked upon and the valuable lessons learned along the way. This final chapter will summarize key takeaways, offer encouragement, and provide additional resources to support you in continuing your healthy lifestyle.

1. Key Takeaways

- *Understanding Your Caloric Needs*: Recognizing your body's caloric needs is the foundation of a balanced diet. A 1500 kcal plan can help you achieve your health goals, whether they involve weight loss, maintenance, or simply improving your overall well-being.

- *Balanced Nutrition*: A balanced diet isn't just about calories; it's about ensuring your body receives the right mix of nutrients—carbohydrates, proteins, fats, vitamins, and minerals. Every meal is an opportunity to nourish your body with the nutrients it needs to thrive.

- *Meal Planning and Preparation*: Successful adherence to a 1500 kcal plan is made easier with thoughtful meal planning and preparation. Having a plan helps you stay on track and prevents impulsive, unhealthy choices.

- *Exercise and Physical Activity*: Integrating regular exercise into your routine enhances the benefits of your 1500 kcal diet. Physical activity supports weight management, boosts energy levels, and improves mental health.

- *Mindful Eating and Healthy Habits*: Mindful eating encourages you to listen to your body's signals and enjoy food without judgment. Combined with healthy lifestyle habits like regular hydration, stress management, and sufficient sleep, you're setting yourself up for long-term success.

- *Consistency and Maintenance*: Achieving your health goals is a journey that requires consistency. The strategies discussed throughout this guide will help you maintain your progress and continue to lead a healthy lifestyle.

2. Embracing the Journey

Maintaining a 1500 kcal diet and a healthy lifestyle is not just about reaching a specific weight or goal—it's about embracing a journey of self-care, well-being, and lifelong health. Here are some final thoughts to keep in mind as you move forward:

- *Celebrate Your Progress*: No matter where you are on your journey, take time to celebrate your achievements. Every small step forward is a victory worth acknowledging.

- *Be Flexible*: Life is dynamic, and so should be your approach to diet and health. Allow yourself the flexibility to adjust your plan as needed, whether it's for special occasions, changing goals, or evolving preferences.

- *Stay Informed*: Nutrition and health are constantly evolving fields. Stay informed by continuing to educate yourself, seeking out credible sources, and being open to new ideas and approaches.

- *Seek Support*: You don't have to go through this journey alone. Whether it's a friend, family member, or a community of like-minded individuals, having support can make a big difference in staying motivated and accountable.

3. Resources for Further Support

To continue your journey, here are some resources you may find helpful:

Books:
1. *"The Mindful Diet: How to Transform Your Relationship with Food for Lasting Weight Loss and Vibrant Health"* by Ruth Wolever, PhD, and Beth Reardon, MS, RD

2. *"How Not to Die: Discover the Foods Scientifically Proven to Prevent and Reverse Disease"* by Dr. Michael Greger

Websites:
1. *MyFitnessPal*: A comprehensive tool for tracking your calories, nutrients, and exercise.

2. *EatRight.org*: The Academy of Nutrition and Dietetics offers a wealth of information on balanced eating and healthy living.

Apps:

1. *Headspace*: Offers guided meditations, including sessions focused on mindful eating and stress reduction.

2. FitOn: A free fitness app offering a variety of workout videos to keep your exercise routine fresh and engaging.

Online Communities:
1. *Reddit* - r/nutrition: A supportive community where you can ask questions and share experiences related to diet and nutrition.

2. *SparkPeople*: An online community focused on healthy living, weight loss, and fitness.

4. Final Encouragement

Remember, the goal is not perfection but progress. Every healthy choice you make contributes to a better, stronger, and more vibrant you. The path to maintaining a balanced diet and a healthy lifestyle may have its challenges, but with the knowledge and tools you've gained from this guide, you are well-equipped to navigate them.

Your health is your most valuable asset—nurture it, protect it, and celebrate it every day.

This concludes "A Guide on Maintaining a Balanced Diet with a 1500 kcal Plan." I hope this guide serves as a helpful companion on your journey to health and wellness. If you need to make any adjustments or add more content, feel free to let me know!

9 798336 052183